SMOOTHIES FOR BETTER HEALTH

SMOOTHIES FOR BETTER HEALTH

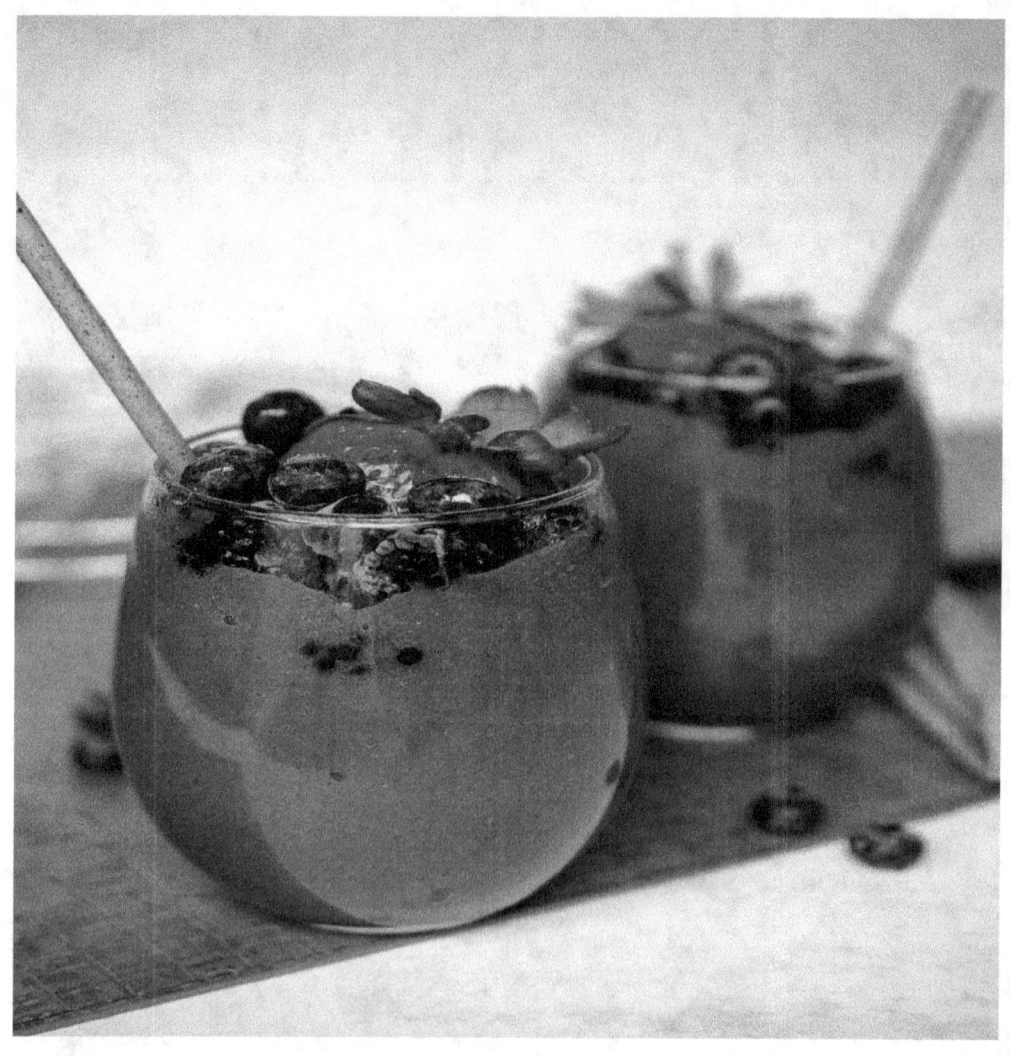

TABLE OF CONTENTS

- INTRODUCTION 3
- CHAPTER 1 5
  - SMOOTHIES FOR BETTER HEALTH 5
- CHAPTER 2 8
  - THE VEGAN SMOOTHIES DIET 8
- CHAPTER 3 11
  - CAN THE SMOOTHIE DIET HELP YOU LOSE WEIGHT? 11
- CHAPTER 4 13
  - GREEN SMOOTHIES - MY KIDS EAT KALE FOR BREAKFAST 13
- CHAPTER 5 16
  - 10 MOST COMMON GREEN SMOOTHIE QUESTIONS 16
- CHAPTER 6 21
  - EASILY ELIMINATE CRAVINGS WHILE ON A GREEN SMOOTHIE DIET 21
- CHAPTER 7 26
  - MAKE STRAWBERRIES ONE OF YOUR NEW FAVORITE SMOOTHIE INGREDIENT 26
- CHAPTER 8 29
  - BUST BELLY FAT: HOW A SMOOTHIE DIET CAN TRIM YOUR TUMMY 29
- CHAPTER 9 33
  - HOW TO LOSE WEIGHT AND BURN FAT DRINKING GREEN SMOOTHIES! 33
- CHAPTER 10 35
  - 33 HEALTHY SMOOTHIE RECIPES FOR WEIGHT LOSS 35
- CONCLUSION 50
  - CHOOSING THE BEST BLENDER FOR YOUR BUDGET 50

INTRODUCTION

A smoothie diet isn't really a diet at all. It's more of a modification to your eating plan. Losing weight has always been at the forefront of modern society. With high-profile celebrity icons being paraded like something in a shop window, we often find ourselves compelled at how these people achieve their gorgeous physiques. Well the truth is that I, just like you are a normal person with work constraints and other commitments which simply take too much time for me to be able to commit myself to attending the gym everyday.

Wouldn't you love to lose weight, manage your five-a-day intake, improve your energy, and improve your skin, hair, and nails? If you answered 'yes' to these questions, then perhaps its time you implemented a smoothie diet into your life.

A smoothie is a mix of various ingredients, mainly fruits and/or vegetables which are blended together to create a great tasting and refreshing 'drink'. However, if we look closely at the ingredients involved in creating a smoothie, you will be amazed at how beneficial a smoothie can be to your body. The U.S. Department of Agriculture Food Pyramid recommends three to five servings of vegetables and two to four servings of fruits per day. Eating just the minimum number of these servings adds up to what is called the "five-a-day." Fewer than 15 percent of Americans eat the minimum five servings of fruits and vegetables a day.

A typical smoothie recipe that I make in the mornings would be one made up of one apple, one banana, one cup of orange juice, a handful of strawberries and two table spoons of natural yoghurt. If you look at the ingredients in that list, I am already consuming the majority of my five-a-day - I am loading my body with goodness and the necessary vitamins and energy I require to have a healthy, balanced body. And I'm doing this whilst enjoying what I'm drinking! Wouldn't you love to experiment with a smoothie diet that actually tastes delicious? Nobody wants ridiculous diet fad ideas such as eating lettuce, or only meat. In the following paragraph I will explain why.

A typical diet will advise you to stick to some sort of eating plan where you are essentially cutting out many of the foods you enjoy and eating fewer portions. Have you ever noticed why there are so many dieting fads? The reason is because they are all temporary fixes for a permanent problem!

Consider this study from the UCLA; "You can initially lose 5 to 10 percent of your weight on any number of diets, but then the weight comes back," said Traci Mann, UCLA associate professor of psychology and lead author of the study. "We found that the majority of people regained all the weight, plus more. Sustained weight loss was found only in a small minority of participants, while complete weight regain was found in the majority. Diets do not lead to sustained weight loss or health benefits for the majority of people."

So why the smoothie diet? I recommend the smoothie diet because essentially it's not really a diet. I'm not asking you to stop eating certain foods, nor am I limiting your quantities. I'm asking you to take the time to integrate smoothies into your lifestyle. Have one for breakfast or lunch, and have one for after your evening meal perhaps? What you will notice is an increase in the amount of energy you have as well as how full you feel. The fibre from the fruit/vegetables is slower to digest, so you will feel fuller for longer. Consume two smoothies a day and you will be literally loading your body with vitamins and minerals, essential to having healthy hair, skin, nails, better eyesight, a stronger immune system and many more beneficial qualities.

All this in addition to the real goal - Losing weight! Yes, you don't need to worry about calorie-counting when it comes to smoothies. Just have fun making them, and have fun drinking them. Fit the smoothie diet around your job; share the fun with your children and most importantly of all, take control of your weight and your future. You will soon notice the pounds drop off and stay off, purely because you will find yourself needing to eat less and because what you are consuming, is naturally good food.

CHAPTER 1

SMOOTHIES FOR BETTER HEALTH

When it comes to our diet, smoothies aren't exactly the first thing that comes to mind when we think about eating healthy. But I'm not talking about chocolate or vanilla smoothies... I'm talking about an all natural, extremely healthy smoothie that is made from greens and other organic products.

Green Smoothies are great, and they are a lot easier than juicing. Many people that start the vegan diet use smoothies as an introduction to the diet. However, green smoothies are great to add to any diet, and as long as you avoid using processed foods, they will provide your body with a wealth of vitamins and minerals that your body needs to function at its best ability.

If you want to add smoothies to your diet purely for health reasons, it is strongly recommended that you make them yourself, and not buy smoothies at restaurants or coffee shops. Generally when these types of businesses make smoothies, they make them for the sole purpose of taste. There are plenty of other ingredients in those smoothies that are not healthy for your body, and in some cases can become detrimental to your health.

Green Smoothies can taste great and you don't need to add any artificial sweeteners. By simply adding any fruit of your choice, you can make it taste sweet. Adding fruit will also give it the creamy feeling that you get when you add milk, without the dairy! Fruits contain soluble fibers, and the best fruits to add to your smoothies are:

1. Pears
2. Bananas
3. Kiwi
4. All Berries

Apples don't really contain soluble fibers, but don't let that stop you from putting it in your smoothie! Adding more fruits only makes it more nutritional, so have a blast and get creative with your smoothies.

Smoothies are beneficial, even if you are not on a diet, and there are in fact numerous health benefits to consuming smoothies daily, including:

1. Increase Your Consumption of Greens and Fruits - Did you know that it is recommended to eat between 4-9 servings of fruit per day? Eating fruits and vegetables can prevent diseases and has even been proven to aid in the prevention of cancer.

2. Great for Weight loss - Smoothies are an amazing way to lose weight naturally and healthily. Try substituting a meal for a healthy well balanced smoothie.

3. More Energy - It has been proven that people who consume all natural smoothies have more energy than those that do not. This is obviously clear, because a smoothie will deliver large amounts of vitamins, minerals and natural sweeteners that will give you that energy boost that you need... without the crash!

4. Increased Fibre Absorption - Green Smoothies are naturally high in fiber because you are using the whole green product and it's not just "juicing" out the water.

5. Chlorophyll - Chlorophyll does everything from enhancing your immune system to helping with the rejuvenation of your body. Chlorophyll has also been known as a "purifier" of the blood.

6. Stops Cravings - Smoothies will stop that craving that you have for junk food. Because smoothies are rich in vitamins, minerals and natural sweeteners, your body will feel very satisfied after consuming a smoothie!

Smoothies are a great addition to any diet, and can be used for more than just healthy living. Smoothies can be used to target certain health goals by combining certain fruits together. It is always recommended to fully educate yourself on the topic before you begin consuming smoothies.

We believe in education over medication, and all natural smoothies definitely align with that belief. However, it is important to know how each fruit will interact with each other and how much protein/fibre/etc. is in each fruit. I'm not saying to keep a chart of stats, but it is good to generally know how much fibre is in each fruit. The worst case scenario is probably a light case of diarrhea, and that would usually be from mixing the wrong fruits together.

If you are considering adding smoothies to your diet then you are already on the right path! Don't let any "nay-sayers", or negative people hold you back from achieving your health goals and start enjoying the health benefits of smoothies today.

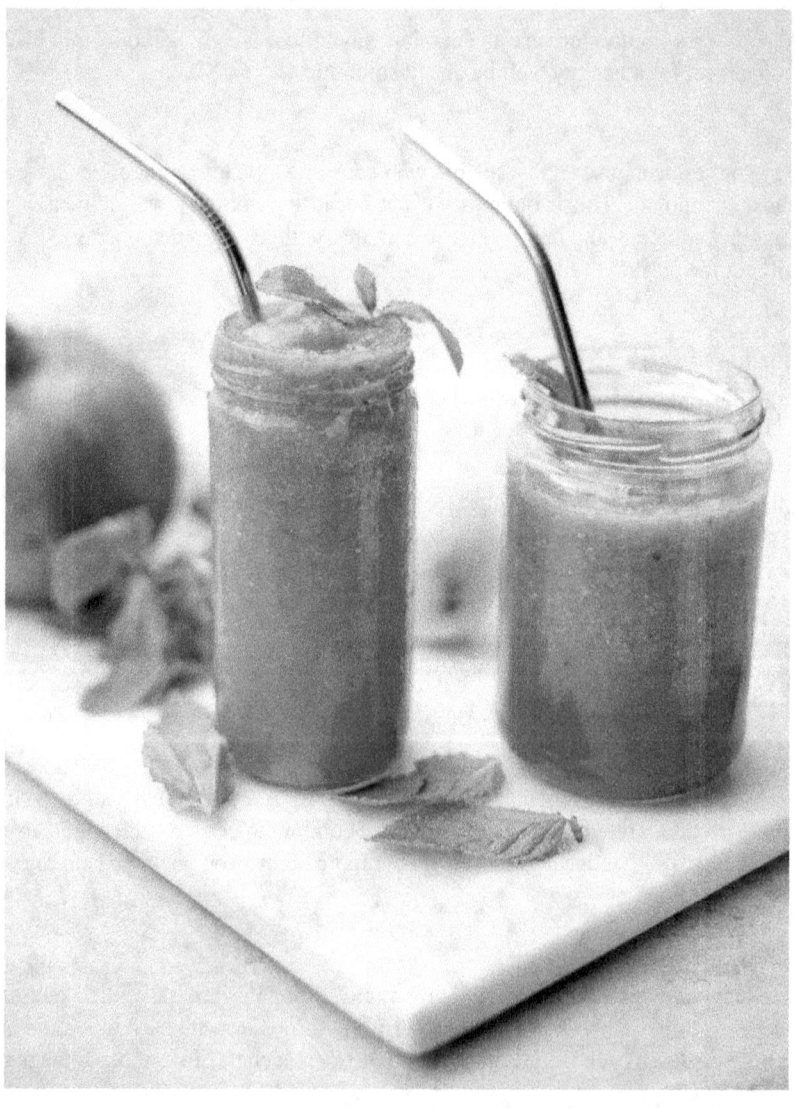

CHAPTER 2

THE VEGAN SMOOTHIES DIET

If you only listened to the commercials you would think that you need to buy special pills or drinks to help you lose weight. Prepackaged drinks, bars, and snacks are sold by the thousands each day to people desperate to lose weight.

The reality is that you can lose weight and gain health from the produce section of your local grocery store. When it comes to burning fat, gaining energy, and feeling great there is no replacement for getting a daily load of fresh fruits and vegetables. The easiest way to do this is with the vegan smoothies diet. Vegan smoothies are so easy to make!

Vegan simple means there is no animal products included. No milk, cheese, or honey. Everything you need was growing on a plant somewhere and is now waiting for you to enjoy. Every day there is a new diet plan being marketed, a new "secret" weight loss formula selling books, or another diet guru on TV. The fads come and go like the weather. Many people are drawn in by these fad diets, promising weight loss results if you just buy all the things they are selling.

The vegan smoothie diet requires no guru, no secret formula, and no expensive meal replacements bars. All you need is a fridge full of fruits and vegetables, a good blender, and a desire to be your best. Rather than some new fad diet, this is the way humans were eating for millions of years. Our ancestors ran on fresh fruits and vegetables in their natural form, and how many overweight, sluggish cavemen do you think survived the harsh conditions?

For some, these fad diets may work at first. Water weight loss or burning of excess fat is common. Unfortunately, it all comes back once you stop the fad dieting. And with it health problems from ingesting unhealthy chemicals and mixes. Instead, a vegan smoothie diet gives your body exactly what it needs. Raw fruits and vegetables. Simple fill up your blender with a few fresh berries, a banana, and a handful of leafy greens. Then mix.

The green smoothie you create may not look good, but it tastes wonderful. The natural sugars found in the fresh fruit is better than the artificial sweeteners found in most foods. And veggie-phobes and take care, you will not taste the greens at all. There are many different ways to create a delicious vegan smoothie, but they all end up the same way: a healthy alternative to fad diets and weight loss lies. When you feed your body what it needs it will easily drop pounds, gain energy, and feel better.

And because this is not a diet, there is no worry about gaining every thing back later. You can continue to enjoy a vegan smoothie once a day, or more, for the rest of your life to continue getting your daily needs without taking away from your life.

What an easy way to lose weight!

The vegan smoothie diet is a simple, fast, and easy solution to weight loss problems. Whether you drink one a day, or three, your body will start to feel better. Drink one each day for breakfast, or as an afternoon snack. Some people love it so much they have a smoothie several times a day.

The incredible nutritional value from one smoothie is far better than most people get in an entire day's worth of meals. Leaving the fruits and vegetables raw means they do not lose precious nutrients from cooking. And blending them up makes it easier for your body to break down and absorb the nutrients there. Unlike with juicing, you are getting the entire thing. Anyone who wants to lose weight without giving up health should try the vegan smoothies diet.

WHAT MAKES SMOOTHIES A VERY SPECIAL KIND OF BEVERAGE?

You may be one of those people who have made the decision to lead a healthier lifestyle. Is that why you are looking for a bit of help? Are you here because you want to know more about how to make delicious and spectacular smoothies?

Smoothies information is so in-demand these days. But, what makes smoothies special when they are just part purée and part fruit drink? They are easy to make, so much so that anyone can prepare one. It takes no special skill to concoct a foamy fruity mix that you can enjoy by yourself or share with people close to you.

What makes smoothies a special type of beverage is that they can be so nutritious that you won't need to take multivitamins and other expensive supplements anymore if you include smoothies in your daily diet. Smoothies are very good for you.

There was a time when smoothies were novelties and specialties offered only in cafes, restaurants, and juice bars. Now you can make them at home. With smoothies information that you can readily access online, anything is possible. If you are new to the smoothie phenomenon, you can learn how to make a handful of basic preparations such as strawberry smoothie, banana smoothie, and mango smoothie. But you should realize that there is a whole new world of smoothies information that you have not yet glimpsed. Allow us to impart a few tips that you can use to make more refreshing, exciting, and very delicious smoothie preparations.

You may already know that the heart of every smoothie preparation is fruit. Some of the most popular fruit choices are banana, pineapple, mango and other tropical fruit. These fruits are not just treats to the taste buds. They make smoothies very special because they contain fiber and essential vitamins and minerals. When preparing smoothies, it is totally up to you whether you want to combine fruit flavors. There is no limit to the number of fruit combinations, and the ratio and proportion of fruit mixing is always a personal decision. This opportunity to exercise creativity is just one of the characteristics that make smoothies a very special kind of beverage.

Many people who need smoothies information want to explore available possibilities on the base component of smoothies. Milk and cream are usual choices, but yoghurt is now becoming a popular alternative. Yoghurt is a good choice because they contain probiotics which are essential in maintaining the health of the gastrointestinal tract. Probiotics help sustain the population of beneficial bacteria in the gut. Yoghurt also contains vitamin D and calcium. If you are concerned about the fat intake, there are low-fat yoghurt preparations that you can opt for. Soy yoghurt is also available if you are a vegan or have lactose intolerance.

When it comes to the choice of sweeteners, there are numerous alternatives to refined sugar. White sugar is linked to a number of health conditions so if you will be preparing smoothies regularly. Some of the better alternatives to refined sugar are honey, nectar, and agave syrup.

There is one last tip that we shall impart to you. Get an excellent blender. Once you have one nothing stands between you and smoothie heaven.

CHAPTER 3

CAN THE SMOOTHIE DIET HELP YOU LOSE WEIGHT?

A lot has been written about the smoothie diet. This information can be found on the internet or in books you can buy at your local book store. Much of this information indicates your weight lose goals can be achieved using this approach. This diet has its pros and cons. Using the proper approach with this wight loss system is key to success and must include a balanced diet.

The smoothie diet includes plenty of vegetables and fruits. The inclusion of these food types is essential to the success of the this type of diet. This diet is low in calories and rich in phytonnutrients. These are chemicals produced by plants. These chemicals are nutrients and are used by plants to protect themselves from damaging environments. Phytonutrients are used by plants to reduce the effects of ultraviolet radiation and pollution, which can cause dangerous free radicals to generate within their cells. Simply put plants produce these nutrients to stay healthy. Phytonutrients are available in supplement form for human consumption, but are best consumed as nutrient-rich foods, such as in a smoothie diet. Having these nutrients contained in a proper smoothie will help reduce inflammation which triggers weight gain.

It should be noted that many food establishments are including smoothies on their menus,or at least the best ingredients to make one. In fact some food establishments are totally dedicated to making and selling these and other healthy drinks, So if your schedule is to busy, you can always visit one of these health food establishments and have a smoothie made for you.

Of course there are some cons with the smoothie diet. This diet can be expensive to implement. You will have to experiment with food to decide which smoothie suits your taste. Although there are many recipes you can find on the internet or in various books, there is no guarantee that the results will taste good. It will take time to find the recipe that not only satisfies your taste buds, but gives you the nutrients you need to make the smoothie diet a success.

Reducing foods such as sugar and saturated fat is key to reducing weight as these are inflammatory foods. Include vegetables, fruits and whole grains which are naturally anti-inflammatory in your diet. This can be achieved with a smoothie diet, however the you will need to have the proper approach to this diet. There are many resources on the internet which can help you with approach.

THE HEALTH BENEFITS OF GREEN SMOOTHIES

Many people find the thought of eating many servings of fruits and vegetables each day to be overwhelming. The thought of eating salads every day or bunches of lettuce and spinach can be enough to discourage people from following a healthier diet. Fortunately, there are a few painless ways to get more leafy greens into your diet without having to feel like a bunny rabbit. Many people who have difficulty eating leafy greens choose to drink them instead in the form of green smoothies. Green smoothies are fruit smoothies that have leafy greens such as spinach or kale blended into them. Getting used to the taste can take a little while, but once you do you can drink the equivalent of an entire salad in the form of a green smoothie.

Drinking green smoothies is an excellent way to increase your vegetable intake. Some common vegetables that can be easily added to smoothies are romaine lettuce, spinach, kale, carrots, celery, and cucumbers. Of course, you should not add all of these at once. Most people who drink green smoothies recommend a ratio of 40% vegetables to 60% fruit to keep it tasting good. If you are just starting out with drinking green smoothies then choose a mild green such as spinach and add a small amount to your smoothie. Once you are more accustomed to the taste you can increase the amount of greens that you are blending.

In addition to increasing your vegetable intake, green smoothies can also help you to eat more fruits. A smoothie may contain a peach, a handful of strawberries, a banana, some blueberries, and an apple. This adds up to at least three or four servings of fruit in one delicious drink. Most people thin their smoothies with 100% fruit juice, although some people choose to use water or milk to get their smoothies to a drinkable consistency.

Besides the benefits of eating more fruits and vegetables, drinking them is also a great way to get more healthy fats into your diet. It is easy to add healthy fats into it without altering the taste or texture of the drink. Adding the meat of an avocado to a green smoothie will significantly increase the healthy fat content without changing the taste. If avocados are hard to find in your area, try adding ground flax seeds to your smoothie. The easiest way to do this is to buy flax seeds whole and grind them yourself a little at a time. Even a few tablespoons of coconut oil added to a smoothie will up the nutritional oomph of your drink significantly.

Many people wonder if drinking green smoothies is better or worse than juicing fruits and vegetables. Although the jury is still out, they have some significant advantages. When you juice, you lose the fruit and vegetable fiber that is part of what makes them so good for you. They allow you to drink all of that fiber easily. It also takes much less fruit to make a green smoothie than it does to make a cup of juice, making green smoothies more economical for many people.

CHAPTER 4

GREEN SMOOTHIES - MY KIDS EAT KALE FOR BREAKFAST

Okay, I admit it...I get some kind of sick pleasure out of saying that I send my kids to school in the morning with a belly full of raw kale or spinach. As I watch them sipping away at their freshly made green smoothies, I pat myself on the back thinking I am such a genius at deception. What parent doesn't want to get more green vegetables into their children's diet? My seven year old daughter cringes at the idea of eating a salad with dinner, but lately I have her happily slurping away at her blueberry smoothies in the morning oblivious to the fact that she is drinking raw spinach. As long as she doesn't actually see the green leaves enter the blender, then it's fine. Blueberries and blackberries work well with her because they cover over the green color, but as far as taste goes, basically any fruit works. My oldest son who is eleven is much more adventurous and will try any concoction I make, regardless of color or texture.

Green smoothies are the easiest place to start for anyone who wants to add more green vegetables into their diets and they are equally appealing to both children and adults. Kids like that they taste good...they think they are getting a treat. Adults like that they taste good too and that they are quick and easy to make. In our busy lives, quick and easy are essential if we intend for a diet or lifestyle change to stick. In my kitchen, the blender remains on the center island counter at all times. A quick rinse and it is ready to be used again. In the morning, I throw in one or two frozen bananas, some frozen berries, two handfuls of whatever greens I have on hand, some water and ice...hit the blend button and breakfast is served. There are no complicated recipes required and experimentation is recommended. My favorite smoothies have been ones I have improvised, not copied out of a recipe book. If I would ever get into the habit of writing down the concoctions I like the best, I may end up with a recipe book of my own!

A full pitcher is enough for my three kids and myself. If it happens to be a particularly popular flavor, I'll give my portion to the kids and make a second batch for myself. This batch I load up with all kinds of supplements. I go easy on the supplements with the kids, because many of them alter the flavor of the smoothie and they won't drink it. Nothing annoys me more than to have to waste all that precious organic produce. Ground flax seed is one supplement that I can add in to theirs without any of them noticing a change in flavor.

Although much of what my kids eat remains outside of my control and I cannot force them to eat something they don't want to, I find the green smoothies to be a win-win situation. The kids love them and I feel good that they are starting the day off with proper nutrients. Over time the more green vegetables they eat, the less they will crave the sugary, processed junk food they are surrounded by at school, their friends' houses and restaurants. I am trying to be patient with their transition to healthier foods. After all, my own transition to a healthier lifestyle has been a journey (several years and counting). There have been many occasions where I have just wanted to throw my hands up in the air and say forget it, I give up (actually I have done that a number of times), but the introduction of green smoothies into our household has given me newfound hope that all is not lost.

Some helpful tips for making green smoothies:

o If you find the flavor too bland with water as the liquid, substitute 1 cup of freshly squeezed orange juice for 1 cup of water. This will give the smoothie a sweeter taste.

o Buy bananas at the store that look very ripe (some brown spots). Peel them and place in a large Ziploc bag in the freezer so you always have them on hand.

o Chop up and freeze your own fruit...buy overly ripe or just do so when you have too much left over.

o Ask your grocer for fruit "seconds"; you may be able to save some money.

o Alternatively, buy bags of frozen organic fruit in the freezer section at your grocery or health foods store. I have found certain brands of strawberries to be way too sour, so try a variety of different brands to find the ones you like the best.

o A very popular supplement with my kids is raw cacao (raw chocolate). Mixed with agave nectar, it adds a rich chocolaty taste to the smoothie. Beware of overdoing it though; raw cacao does contain caffeine. Carob powder is another choice that does not contain caffeine.

o If you end up with too much of a batch, store the remainder in the refrigerator covered with saran wrap for an after-school snack. Smoothies and grapes are a much better choice than cookies and milk.

o Get the kids involved in the fruit choices; they are much more likely to eat something they have helped to create.

o To make a smoothie thicker, add more ice. To thin it out add more liquid (water, nut milk, or orange juice depending on recipe).

o To sweeten a smoothie, add a couple Tablespoons of raw agave nectar or raw honey.

For those of you who feel more comfortable following a recipe, I am including a couple different variations here, but please experiment on your own after you have made these. If you come up with something really great, let me know about it! (Feel free to use the greens interchangeably...you really can't taste them).

Blueberry Kale:

1 cup frozen blueberries

2 frozen bananas

2 handfuls chopped kale

2 cups water (or 1 cup water and 1 cup freshly squeezed orange juice)

handful of ice

Optional: 1 T ground flax seed

Grape Fig Cleanser: (grapes are very cleansing and detoxifying)

3 cups grapes (purple or green)

3-4 black mission figs

2 handfuls chopped spinach

2 T agave nectar

2 cups water

1 cup ice

Optional: 1 T ground flax seed

Peach Almond Smoothie:

1 cup frozen peaches

2 frozen bananas

2 handfuls chopped swiss chard

2 T raw almond butter

2 cups water

¼ cup agave nectar

1 tsp vanilla

Optional: 1 T ground flax seed

CHAPTER 5

10 MOST COMMON GREEN SMOOTHIE QUESTIONS

QUESTION: How much green smoothie do you recommend I drink daily?

ANSWER: In the beginning people tend to drink more green smoothies, sometimes up to two gallons per day depending on how acidic their body pH is. After several months the quantity goes down to 1-2 quarts per day.

QUESTION: Do I have to make fresh green smoothie several times per day?

ANSWER: Smoothies can stay in the refrigerator for 2-3 days, but fresh is best. As soon as a smoothie is warmed to room temperature, it should be consumed.

QUESTION: How much greens does one really need? I generally consume a head of lettuce. Do you think this is enough?

ANSWER: One needs fewer greens in the form of green smoothies than in the form of salad, because blended greens assimilate several times more thoroughly then chewed greens. I estimate that if you prefer to eat greens as a salad, you should consume at least two bunches of greens (or 6 packed cups) per day. If you drink your greens in blended form, then one bunch (3 packed cups) will be sufficient per day.

People who have an acidic pH balance in their body could benefit from consuming up to 80% greens in their diet. When they reach a stage of balance, they will notice that they want less greens and less green smoothies, but they will enjoy them more than ever.

QUESTION: It seems you talk about having an entire bunch of chard, or other greens, daily. Yet in your recipes, a smoothie only has 3-5 leaves from an entire bunch. Are you having more than 1 smoothie a day?

ANSWER: The goal is to eventually consume more greens in the smoothie than fruit. However, many of us are not used to consuming large amounts of greens. Also many don't have adequate hydrochloric acid to digest greens. For this reason, I recommend starting with more fruity green smoothies and slowly using more and more greens. As the body finds out the many benefits of greens, it becomes very excited and starts craving greener smoothies. Experiment with what amount of greens you find palatable and gradually add more greens so that you work up to the equivalent of one average-sized bunch of greens per day.

It is possible that you will start with a fruity green smoothie and progress to extremely green smoothies. Yet, there will be another change later. As you keep consuming green smoothies on a regular basis for many months, you will eventually reduce the total amount of green smoothies that you consume daily.

This happens because the assimilation of nutrients increases and the body can get more nutrients from less smoothies, your body satisfies the most urgent needs for nutrients, it also becomes more alkaline and doesn't need as much greens as before. Please remember to keep rotating your greens for variety!

QUESTION: How long should I blend my ingredients to make the green smoothie?

ANSWER: I usually blend my greens and fruits for 30-45 seconds. I always start on the low speed and turn it up to high.

QUESTION: I cant afford to buy a Vitamix or a Blendec, can I use a regular blender?

ANSWER: The reason it is recommended to use a high speed blender for making green smoothies is because the cell walls are easily broken up and the machine will last. You can use a regular blender to make your smoothies, it is better than not making any smoothies at all, however the greens may not be broken to a creamy consistency and the blender motor will probably burn out quickly.

QUESTION: What kind of blender do I need to make green smoothies?

ANSWER: You may use any blender to make smoothies, however I recommend using the most powerful blender you can find, 1000 watts or more. If you don't have a powerful blender, you can still make green smoothies and benefit from them, but you will have to chop your ingredients into smaller pieces, blend for longer periods of time, and to put up with some chunks in your smoothie. A smoothie prepared in a high-speed blender is smooth in consistency, and will be assimilated better by the body. For those who live in the United States I recommend any model of the Vita-Mix blender.

If you live outside of the United States, I recommend another high-speed blender called, Blendtec, which is priced reasonably for international sales.

QUESTION: Can I freeze smoothies or will they be less nutritious frozen?

ANSWER: I have never frozen my greens, but if I lived in a northern country and had, for example, a large harvest of spinach, I would freeze it and use it over time. Frozen greens will still be more nutritious than cooked greens. However, if you have access to fresh greens, they are significantly more nutritious and tastier than frozen.

QUESTION: Since I started drinking green smoothies my stool became green. Is it normal?

ANSWER: When the stomach acid is low, one may find pieces of undigested food in the stool and color of it may reflect the color of the food consumed such as red from beets, green from green smoothie, etc. After daily consumption of green smoothies, the body receives plenty of nourishment and the level of stomach acid begins to normalize. Eventually you will always observe the same stool despite of your food intake. Normal stool should be light-brown in color, odorless, well formed and not sticking to the toilet. It leaves the body easily with no straining or discomfort.

QUESTION: Why is it so important that humans model their diet after chimpanzees? From my understanding, they only live an average of 50 years. They are usually riddled with parasites too.

ANSWER: Chimpanzees are genetically the closest creatures to humans. They share 99.4% of genes with humans. That is why, unfortunately, chimpanzees are used for medical research. However, chimpanzees have often demonstrated such a strong immunity, that doctors were not able to infect them with HIV or hepatitis C. In my book, I brought up the point that instead of making chimps ill with human diseases, researching how they are able to stay healthy may reveal immensely valuable information on human health. In captivity, chimpanzees do live much longer than in the wild because they are guarded against accidents and environmental dangers.

Chimpanzees are not only healthy, but have the ability to intuitively find and use healing herbs. Scientists from the Jane Goodall Institute described in their research that chimpanzees are familiar with natural ways of parasite control by eating medicinal herbs. On the other hand, any colonic therapist will tell you how so many humans are laden with all kinds of parasites.

THE BEST TIME OF THE DAY FOR A GREEN SMOOTHIE

Juicing and blending - the terms are often used interchangeably, but there is striking difference between the two. The difference is in the manner in which each is made. When fruits and vegetables are juiced, the liquid is extracted and the indigestible fiber is discarded, however when fruits and vegetables are blended to make a smoothie, they are served with the fibrous material.

This basic difference is the reason why juices can be had at any time during the day but smoothies cannot. Green smoothies with all their fibrous material are harder to digest. Hence, nutritionists and health experts advise against having one later in the day. The best time is also determined on the basis of how you have it - as a substitute for a meal or combined with a whole meal.

Morning - The Best Time

A green smoothie for breakfast is seen as the best option. There are several reasons for it. First, an empty stomach ensures better absorption of nutrients and minerals packed in the veggie-fruity blend. Second, as they take longer time to digest, they keep you felling full for a longer period of time and prevent binge eating. Green smoothies are not high in calories but are a dense energy source. Thus, it is a great way to break the morning fast and keeps energy levels from dipping.

A Good Substitute for Lunch

A green smoothie is a healthy replacement for a lunch meal, particularly when you are at work. Lunch breaks tend to be very short and there's no time to eat a proper meal in peace. People either opt for frozen packaged foods gorge on fast food available at the cafeteria. This is where you can have a green smoothie. You can finish it soon. Not only this, it is convenient to carry to work. Besides, small-size portable blenders allow one to make a fresh blend of fruits and vegetables in a minute. Make sure you have a glass big enough - 32 oz or a litre as it is necessary to provide your body with an adequate amount of calories.

After a Workout

A workout - a hard, laborious one - literally whets your appetite. As the body is depleted of energy, it craves for food. Many drink protein shakes and artificially sweetened juices after an exercise session. Instead, you can prepare and have a green smoothie after a workout session. As the heart rate is already elevated, the body will break down foods faster to convert food into energy for the body.

When you start drinking green smoothies, don't go overboard with them. If you have a smoothie for breakfast, do not have one for lunch and dinner too because it has been touted as a healthy alternative. The body requires all the food groups in a balanced amount and going on all-smoothie diet is as good as a crash or fad diet that starves the body. As far as dinner time is concerned, though we wouldn't recommend it, you can have a tall glass of green smoothie instead of your meal.

CHAPTER 6

EASILY ELIMINATE CRAVINGS WHILE ON A GREEN SMOOTHIE DIET

The Proverbial Medical Disclaimer

I'd like to start of by stating that this information is just my opinion based on the information I have read from expert authors and from the 10+ years living and eating the way I have on a daily basis. Couple that with my twice a year blood work that reveals no deficiencies, I feel this information is valid and very valuable. Perhaps it works just for me, my genetic makeup and my body type, I can't say for sure. However, just like cigarette smoke could probably affect each one of us with varying degrees of health negatives, the green smoothie diet, I feel, can affect each one of us with varying degrees of health positives. Try it for yourself, after you speak with your natural, or other, health practitioner first of course.

Cut Your Finger And It Will Usually Be Healed In A Short Time

The body is designed to heal itself right? Then why is it that so many people are sick? Perhaps it is in inaccurate statement that the body is truly designed to heal itself? No! The problem is that we a) do not give it the sufficient amount of tools, by way of diet for the most part, it needs to heal itself and b) we bombard it with things that hinder the functionality of the limited tools that we do provide it.

Living On Mars

Another possibility that may seem a bit far fetched and from another planet is that perhaps our beliefs truly do control our lives. For example if we truly, without a doubt, 100% believe that smoking and eating anything that we want contributes to good health, then it will. That's the theory anyway and I have seen that hold true on smaller scales, like placebos for example, but it's a difficult concept for most people to wrap their minds around so to speak, so let's come back to Earth and finish this up.

You Are What You Eat

Here's a bold statement. One that a lot of people won't like to hear, and one that is just MY opinion and not to be construed as advice. I feel, we, as humans, don't need to consume meat to survive. That's right, the plant kingdom has everything we need to survive and thrive. What about Vitamin D? Get some sun. Plus there are some algaes I believe that provide a source of Vitamin D. What about Vitamin B12? Sure, B12 is abundant in meat, granted, and besides some forms of algae, there may not be a source of B12 in the plant kingdom. However, it is suggested that one of two things may be going on in our favor. First, it is suggested that B12 will recycle itself in the colon so it does not need to be ingested. And another school of thought is that the body will manufacture B12 on its own using other resources that are provided by diet. Who knows for sure, but I'm not deficient in Vitamin B12 myself and I don't eat meat anymore.

The Best Diet Going

I'm a big advocate of raw foods. The suggestion that heating food above a certain temperature destroying much needed enzymes that are important for digestion makes sense to me. Further, it is suggested that to get the most out of our food we must chew it until it disappears. Our body has troubles handling big chunks of food. Also, I strongly believe that we can survive and thrive off of a diet of mostly fruits and dark green leafy vegetables, with the occasional healthy fats. Healthy fats in the form of avocados, soaked nuts and seeds is all I consume.

My goal each day is to eat plenty of raw ripened fruits and greens. The best way as far as I'm concerned, in order to consume enough and to help my body with digestion is to drink green smoothies throughout the day. Finally, I am creating a body that has ALL the tools that it needs to heal itself and give me the energy, mental clarity and vitality that I need to get through my day.

One Major Hurdle: Cravings

Some people worry about the green smoothies tasting bad. That's before they try them. Others worry about losing the "social" aspect of eating. Get over that or be creative or stay sick OK? Another hurdle is cost. Eating unhealthy is cheap that's for sure. But we're just talking about produce here for the most part. If you can't afford to grow your own or to buy organic at first, don't. Eventually, as you heal and feel better, if you are like me, you will start to become more productive and more energetic which could eventually lead to the desire and motivation to grow a garden or even earn more money to buy organic foods. I'm not kidding!

Another hurdle for some, and a big one for me was fighting unhealthy cravings. Just like a person addicted to drugs or alcohol must go through a detox to heal, we essentially have to do the same thing. Our cells are made up of stuff from the food that we have consumed in the past. The body may crave more of the same unhealthy foods that contribute to the contents of the individual, sick cells in our body. For drug detoxes, often times, sauna therapy is used to sweat the drugs out of the system. That generally helps eliminate the physical drug cravings allowing the individual a better chance of staying sober. For us, improving our eating will trigger the elimination of toxic foods as well which can be naturally removed in stool, sweat and urine. However, we still might crave those foods while some of the toxic elements in our cells are still present.

I, myself, have found that immediately after having the first drink of my green smoothie the cravings for greasy foods, meat, sweets, salt, etc started to subside. After I was done drinking the smoothie, the cravings were gone completely and I'd be content. The problem then was that the cravings would come again as I became hungry. What I did was make sure I was on top of it and have a green smoothie ready and waiting before the cravings would reoccur, or shortly after they reared their ugly heads. The unhealthy cravings eventually subsided for good as I cleaned out my body. Suddenly I began to crave greens instead!

Be Proactive

How many small kitchen appliances do you see collecting dust? People use them once and since they don't like to clean them, they avoid using them again. Please don't attach that negative feeling to this process and to your life saving smoothie blender! What works for me is, I make a smoothie, pour it into a mason jar, and then immediately rinse out the lid and the blender and set it on a dish rack to dry. It's then ready to go for the next time around. Just take it apart to clean at the end of the day, not for each use! Forget that noise! Plus, give your jars a good rinse after drinking to avoid having to scrub them later. You may be eating a lot of smoothies at first as your body heals. Eventually, though, you'll likely require less and less, but still maintain the same vitality, energy and ideal weight!

TOP 5 MOST HELPFUL TIPS FOR THE GREEN SMOOTHIES DIET FIRST TIMER

If you're a green smoothies diet first timer, here are some helpful tips you can follow to help you get started:

1. Start your day with a glass of healthy smoothie

Whether you eat breakfast at 6 am or just before noon, start your day with a glass of fruit and vegetable smoothie. This is because the nutrients that smoothies contain work best on an empty stomach. Also, vitamins and minerals are absorbed by the body faster when it's hungry.

2. Make sure that your smoothies contain the complete set of macronutrients

It is important to make sure that each glass of your smoothie contain carbohydrates, fat and protein. While all fruits and vegetables contain good amount of carbohydrates, adding a few sources of healthy fat and protein will make your drink nutritionally complete. Avocados and coconut oil are excellent sources of healthy fats while raw eggs, nuts and seeds provide the protein you need.

3. Practice healthy eating

While drinking a glass or two of simple green smoothies a day provide the body with plenty of health benefits, you shouldn't rely in that fact alone. A green smoothies diet is only meant to support your healthy lifestyle - be sure to consume balanced and nutritious meals along with your smoothies. It also helps to have a good daily exercise routine to keep your heart healthy.

4. Use a variety of vegetables for your healthy smoothies

While not everyone is fond of eating vegetables, experts advise to use more vegetables in your smoothies than fruits. Mixing up your greens allows you to gain different kinds of essential vitamins and minerals. Don't forget to use leafy greens such as spinach, kale, collard greens, parsley, cabbage and lettuce in your simple green smoothies - these nutrition powerhouses will keep your health in check.

5. Be creative with your fruit and vegetable smoothie combinations

While on a green smoothies diet, it is vital that you don't get tired of the same taste over and over again - this will only push you to lose interest in the diet. Considering the appropriate fruit and vegetable combinations, mix and match different types of produce to achieve different tastes. Use a different smoothie base each time - choose from purified water, different types of milk or different flavors of fresh juices and yogurt. You can also choose to add nuts and seeds for varied texture of your smoothies.

As mentioned above, anyone can go through a green smoothies diet provided that healthy eating is practiced a good exercise routine is practiced daily. Without these two, simple green smoothies won't be able to work their magic in your body.

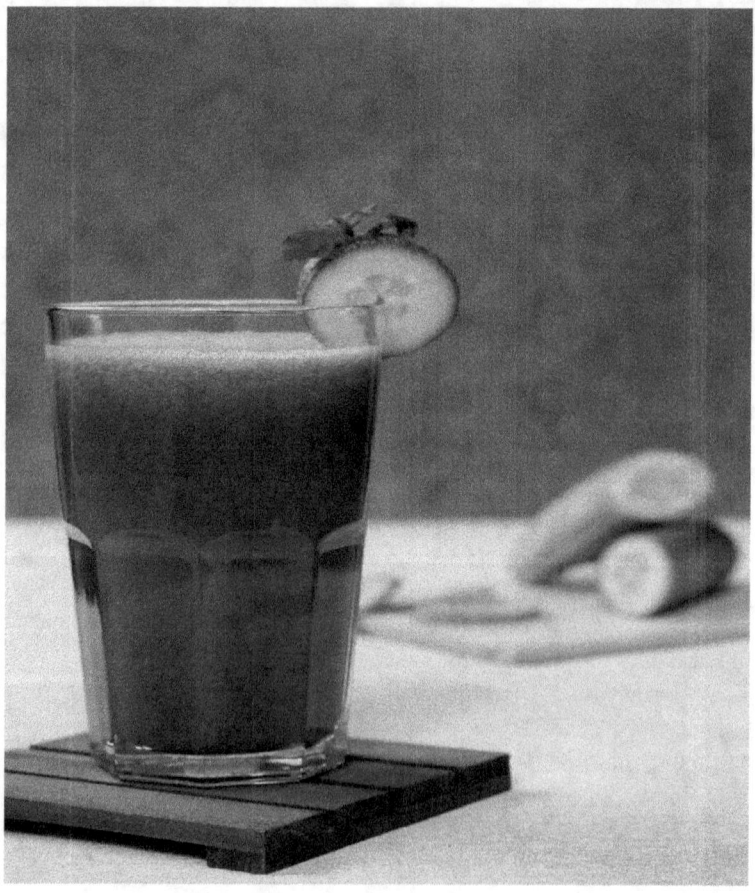

CHAPTER 7

MAKE STRAWBERRIES ONE OF YOUR NEW FAVORITE SMOOTHIE INGREDIENT

Strawberries may be small, but the vibrant color and heart-shaped appearance already give people the idea that it is a healthy, nutritious, and sumptuous fruit that have numerous health benefits when eaten regularly.

Why are strawberries such fantastic fruits? Well, for starters, strawberries taste of summer breeze and sunny days. But that's not the reason why strawberries must be a regular part of the diet. They also have low calorie content, and are fat-free, cholesterol-free, and sodium free as well. That's why strawberries come highly recommended by health professionals.

The health benefits of strawberries have been recognized since Roman times when they were first cultivated. Strawberries are plump and succulent fruits that work their magic in the human body. Your favorite strawberry smoothies recipe also has a cardioprotective effect, helps protect against cancer, increases good cholesterol levels in the bloodstream, and lowers blood pressure.

What makes strawberries an awesome fruit? It's all about the nutrient content. A strawberry smoothies recipe is good for you not just because it is sure to taste wonderful. Rather, every glass that you will consume is filled with fiber and vitamins, but most especially anti-oxidants.

Today, strawberries are among the top 50 foods in the world with the highest antioxidant content. As a matter of fact, strawberries exceed most foods in this respect, being ranked 4th amongst fruits in antioxidant content. Only raspberries, cranberries, and blackberries ranked higher. But if you want to get a full dose of antioxidants, you can easily incorporate these berries into your favorite strawberry smoothies recipe.

Strawberries are also rich in potassium, manganese, and especially Vitamin C. Did you know that a serving of strawberries have a higher Vitamin C content than a whole orange fruit?

Strawberry fans know that bit of trivia and now that you do, you'll definitely end up a strawberry convert. These days, strawberries are given the label, "superfood" and strawberry smoothies recipe are some of the most popular search items around. Why? It's because smoothies have become the trendy medium to consume nutritious fruits and vegetables. Moreover, strawberry smoothies are so refreshing and unequivocally versatile that people have forsaken cocktails to favor this healthier alternative.

What makes smoothies the best types of beverage around is their versatility. The sky is the limit when choosing ingredients. There may be scores of recipes online, but each and every person can make his or her own strawberry smoothies recipe and not even smoothie experts can say that they did wrong or chose too many or too little ingredients. It's all about personal taste and preference.

Do you have your own strawberry smoothies recipe? If so, you can stick to it and enjoy your own preparations. But if you want to explore the creations of other smoothie enthusiasts, a quick Internet search will surely reveal a lot of exciting and unique ideas that you can take inspiration from.

So, stop thinking about strawberries as delicate and perishable fruits that will immediately bruise at even the slightest touch. It is good to always have a bowl of strawberries in your home. They make great snacks and when made into smoothies, you get a taste of summer and a glass of refreshing drink that's very good for your health.

STRAWBERRY BANANA SMOOTHIES YOUR KIDS WILL LOVE

Guess what the most popular smoothie is. If you were to ask a bunch of different people what their favorite was, what do you think would come up high on the list? Most likely, it would be strawberry banana smoothies.

Something this popular has to taste great! So it's a good time to follow the trend and add your own unique spin to the concoction.

What is it about strawberry and banana that makes the combo so popular? Banana is a creamy and mellow-sweet fruit, for one thing.

Strawberries are of course very sweet, but they are also quite tart and rich with passion. They go perfectly with the sweet and mellower bananas.

Strawberry banana smoothies usually include a mixture of the fruits along with ice and milk. That's a delicious recipe as it is, but you can still find ways to make it even better.

The real beauty behind smoothie recipes is that you can use almost any combination of fruits you can think of, blend them together, and come out with something that tastes fantastic.

Here's a quick tip: Try tossing in some blueberries when you're mixing up strawberry banana smoothies. This will add a subtle layer of flavor to die for.

This is an excellent option for smoothies if you're having trouble getting all the antioxidants you need every day.

Oh, and chocolate tastes wonderful in smoothies that contain strawberries and bananas. Ever tasted bananas or strawberries dipped in chocolate?

If you've experienced this, you know how delicious this combo is. So, try mixing in some chocolate ice cream or yogurt with your smoothie.

But if this is going to be part of a smoothie diet, you'll want to make it as healthy as possible. As odd as this sounds, you should try adding chard or kale to your smoothie, since this will give you an even better dose of vitamins.

So what you get is a wonderful drink that tastes of strawberries and bananas, but you'll still get your healthy greens.

Just have fun with it, okay around, and see what you get. It won't be long before you're coming up with your own concoctions of strawberry and banana. If you make this a regular part of your diet, your doctor will be amazed by your health.

Finding good smoothie recipes is the best way to get started. Use them as a jumping point to learn all about what you can do with delicious, healthy smoothies.

CHAPTER 8

BUST BELLY FAT: HOW A SMOOTHIE DIET CAN TRIM YOUR TUMMY

As another mother, beer-drinker, or probably any other person would attest - one of the hardest places to lose weight in is the belly. Even if one is on a diet, belly fat doesn't really go away that easily. But ab crunches and smaller meal portions aside, there is actually a way to trim tummy fat that isn't as strenuous ab-intensive exercises or as expensive as cosmetic surgery.

A smoothie diet is a great weight loss solution but this liquid diet weight loss program can also be used to specifically bust belly fat. Here are two smoothie diet weight loss solutions you can try to get rid of your gut.

Pure Smoothie Diet for 3 Days

Starving yourself just to lose weight isn't healthy so a liquid diet weight loss regimen is a good way to cut the calories but still get the nutrition you need, especially from fruit or vegetable smoothies.

If you want to lose weight (and your belly) fast, consume nothing but smoothies and water for 3 days. But take note, some smoothies especially those from restaurants still contain a lot of calories so a homemade smoothie diet is still the best solution.

Make sure your smoothies are made from fresh and organic fruit and vegetables. Keep your fruit and vegetable selections as colorful as possible - peaches, bananas, cucumber, and spinach are good smoothie diet options.

However, since you can't consume solid food for up to 3 days, make sure you take up to 16 helpings of fruit and vegetable smoothies a day as well as 16 glasses of water or more.

Just make sure you don't stay on this smoothie diet beyond the 3 days or take fruit or vegetable juice as a substitute - it isn't healthy to just live on smoothies and water. This is a great liquid diet weight loss solution that can help you get rid of belly fat but you still have to eat solid food to be fit and healthy.

Belly-Busting Smoothie Diet Ingredients

Now being on a liquid diet (and eating solid food) isn't enough to facilitate weight loss, much less get rid of your gut.

There are some ingredients you can incorporate into your smoothie diet to improve your liquid diet weight loss. Here are some of them:

Protein. Add milk, yogurt, and whey or protein powder into your smoothie because protein is essential for weight loss. This would help you feel fuller as well and keep you from eating more than you need.

Fiber. Fiber rich food such as oatmeal, nuts, fruits, flax seed, and wheat germ can improve bowel movement, prevent constipation, and a bloated belly. Apple skins, oranges, and vegetables are a great source of fiber.

Calcium. Studies show that calcium-rich food like low-fat or non-fat cheese or milk can reduce a person's risk for obesity and heart disease.

To optimize this liquid diet, avoid artificial sweeteners like white sugar, honey, brown sugar, or even maple syrup. These just add unnecessary calories with little nutritional value. Fresh fruits are natural sugar sources so use these instead in your weight loss diet.

7 EASY, DELICIOUS WAYS TO GET MORE RAW FOOD INTO YOUR DIET

It's in the newspaper, on TV and over the Internet: if you want to reduce your risk of developing various diseases, you need to eat more raw food. You know you should, but your conception of raw food is a bunch of lettuce and maybe a carrot stick, and you would like to have a little more taste to your meals than that.

Today, let me help you change that conception. Most raw foods pack a lot flavor and nutrients. And incorporating them into your eating routine is simple. To get you started on discovering the joy of eating raw food, try some of the following ideas.

1. Drink a green smoothie for breakfast (or anytime). You know what a smoothie is-fresh and frozen fruit blended together to make a sweet, tasty drink. A green smoothie is the same, only with a handful of raw greens added to it. Start by trying spinach or leaf lettuce, as they are the more mild-tasting greens (spinach will actually make your smoothie sweeter). The more bitter greens such as romaine lettuce and kale require either more sweet fruit added to the smoothie, or an acquired taste.

2. Snack on celery sticks or cucumber slices with raw nut butter. The vegetables take little time to wash and cut up. You can make your own raw nut butter by whirling raw nuts in a food processor, or buy raw nut butter online or at your local health food store.

3. Eat raw fruit for dessert. If you're addicted to having something sweet after a meal, try some grapes, berries, or dates instead of the usual processed sweets. You could even get real adventurous and try some papaya, which will aid in the digestion process.

4. Eat a large, colorful salad once a day. Make it with at least two cups of lettuce, some chopped non-green bell pepper, and other raw veggies that you enjoy. Top it with your favorite healthy salad dressing.

5. Serve sauerkraut with red meat. I don't mean the conventional kind of sauerkraut that consists of cooked cabbage soaked in vinegar. I mean sauerkraut made of raw cabbage that was fermented at room temperature using salt and/or whey. If you have time, you can make your own. Otherwise, health food stores (and some conventional grocery stores in the health food refrigerated section) carry lacto-fermented sauerkraut in the refrigerated section, near the dairy products. The only ingredients on the label should be cabbage and salt, and perhaps whey.

6. Top your vegetables with sprouts. Growing your own sprouts in a jar is easy and takes little time. Seeds from alfalfa, clover, and broccoli are ready to be eaten in six or seven days, and add nutrition as well as enzymes to a meal. Put a handful on your steamed vegetables or a salad, add some dressing, and dig in!

7. Replace cheese made from pasteurized milk with cheese made from raw milk. The raw milk cheese is healthier and can be found at any grocery store. Similarly, you may consider replacing one cooked meat meal a week with sushi.

Now you have a good starting place to begin to incorporate more raw foods into your diet without sacrificing taste. Bon appetit!

Emily Jacques is a natural health nut, mother, and online wellness coach. Want to improve your health and enhance your sense of well-being? What better way than to receive coaching every week from someone who wants to see you excel in every area of life!

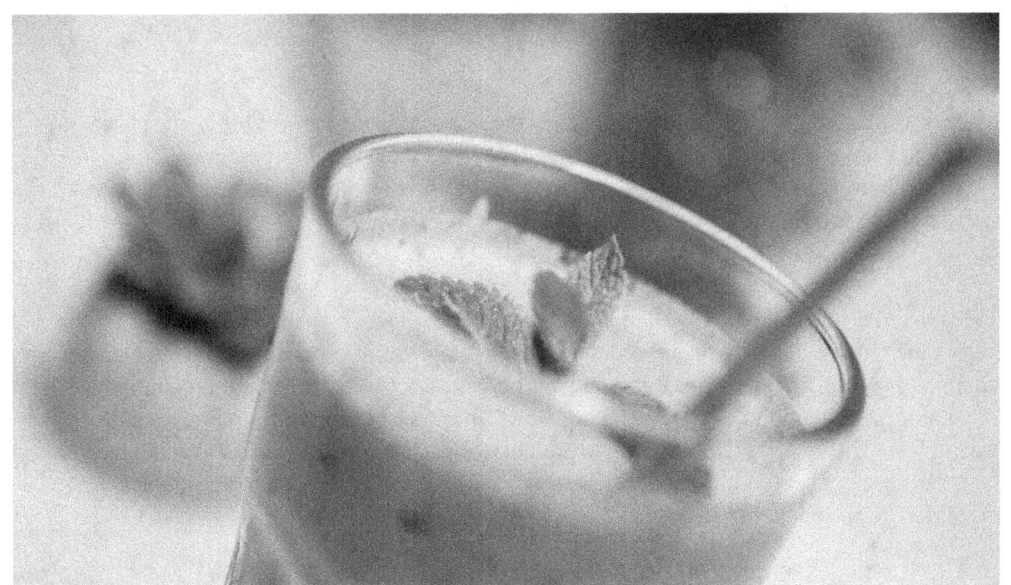

CHAPTER 9

HOW TO LOSE WEIGHT AND BURN FAT DRINKING GREEN SMOOTHIES!

The weight loss industry would like to sell you special herbs and vitamins that they claim can burn fat and help you to lose weight without dieting or exercise. They prefer that you continue to buy their expensive weight loss meal replacements than for you to make your own Green Smoothies.

When it comes to an easy and rapid way to lose weight and burn fat without hunger, drinking Green Smoothies is one of the best ways to achieve your weight loss goals. Green Smoothies are so easy to make! Green Smoothies also taste great and not only will they help you lose weight and burn fat but drinking Green Smoothies can help protect you from many diseases.

It seems that every other month there is a new weight loss diet plan, program or book on the market that promises you can easily lose all of the weight you want if you will just buy and use their special fat burning herbs, vitamin supplements, meal replacement powders or diet book.

More often than not, most of those who do try the latest, greatest fad diet programs instead of drinking Green Smoothies will initially lose a few pounds and maybe even knock off a few inches of fat from their waistline due to the reduced caloric intake most of these programs require you to follow.

That's because in the short term all diets and weight loss reduction plans that require you to reduce the volume of food you are accustomed to eating will work to a certain degree and cause your body to drop a kilo or two. But then your body instinctively goes into protection mode because it perceives itself as starving and it slows your metabolism down to prevent further weight loss. Then when you finally grow tired of always being hungry because you have not been eating enough to feel full and stay hunger free you soon discover that the slightest increase in calories results in rapid weight gain.

Drinking Green Smoothies is a very delicious and highly nutritious and easy way to burn fat, lose weight and fool your body into speeding up your metabolism while decreasing your daily intake of calories all without ever having to feel hungry.

A Green Smoothie Diet is a great tasting way to lose weight and burn fat!

Talk about an easy weight loss program. This simple, fast and easy solution to weight loss will not only help burn fat and melt the pounds away reducing your BMI (Body Mass Index) but at the same time it will fill you up and deliver a flood of nutrients and antioxidants to your cells without having to purchase any expensive artificial supplements.

All you have to do is start your day off by making and drinking "Green Smoothies" that can fill you up while tricking your body into thinking its consuming more because of all the high quality natural nutrition and antioxidants its been craving for but can't get from a standard American (SAD) diet.

Don't confuse making Green Smoothies with juicing, You'll make these delicious energy boosters in your kitchen blender and once you try them and discover how super great you'll feel after drinking them you will want to make them a part of your weight loss routine.

If you want to lose weight try drinking Green Smoothies. You'll never again have to feel hungry and deprive your body of the real food and nutrition it needs. Try the "Green Smoothie Diet" for easy weight loss. Its free and tastes great too!

Imagine, now you can lose weight and burn fat without buying any weight loss pills or supplements because you can lose weight by making your own Green Smoothies whenever you want. But instead of drinking Green Smoothies to just burn fat and lose weight, why not drink them because doing so will make you feel great and live longer!

CHAPTER 10

33 HEALTHY SMOOTHIE RECIPES FOR WEIGHT LOSS

The beauty of adding smoothies to your daily meal plans is how versatile they are. Depending on your mood, you can whip up a really sinfully sweet delight for an afternoon treat or after dinner dessert, or you can create a delicious low calorie high nutrition smoothie that works great for breakfast or a snack.

What follows here are some very good smoothie recipes from both the low calorie and the "not so much" camps. Hope you enjoy them

1. Banana Split Smoothie:

This recipe is a good example of a smoothie that isn't focused on being low calories. Even though it isn't too caloric if you don't use the vanilla ice cream, the honey does add some calories. Nevertheless, this is a really good dessert smoothie.

2 bananas

8 oz. crushed pineapple, without the juice

1 1/4 cup of milk (low-fat if desired)

1/2 cup strawberries (frozen or fresh)

2 tbs. honey

6 ice cubes

(optional): 1 scoop of vanilla ice cream

Add one or more of these optional garnishes to complete the Banana Split experience!

Whipped cream topping

Dark chocolate syrup

Maraschino cherries

Preparation

put the bananas, crushed pineapple, milk, strawberries and honey in your smoothie blender. Blend everything until smooth, with no lumps. Begin to add the ice slowly while still blending until the mix is the preferred consistency. Serve in a chilled glass and add the garnishes of your choice. The result: a banana split in a glass!

In the other camp are those that use smoothies as a "green" drink and swear by their detoxification properties. Because the best smoothies are made with fresh fruits and fresh vegetables, they act as a natural detox program with the benefit of providing a great deal of required vitamins, minerals, and other nutrients at the same time.

Four "detox" smoothie recipes:

2. Grapefruit "detox" smoothie

1 1/2 cups grapefruit juice, freshly squeezed is preferred

3/4 cup of sliced pineapple

1/4 cup of pineapple juice (this will sweeten it up nicely)

1 cup plain low-fat yogurt

2 cups ice

Optional: feel free to add a scoop of ice cream for an even sweeter taste.

3. Lime and Mango "detox" smoothie

1 mango, without peel or pit

1 lime, without seeds or skin

1/4 to 1/2 cup of fresh cilantro, chopped

4 to 6 ounces of filtered water

4. Lime and Lemon "detox"x Smoothie

1/2 lemon, without seeds or skin

1/2 lime, also without seeds or skin

2 bananas, peeled

juice from 1 large orange

Pineapple "detox" smoothie

2 cups filtered water

1/4 medium pineapple

2 medium bananas, peeled

1 orange, peeled

1/2 head romaine lettuce

5. The Tropical Dream

This delicious fruit and vegetable smoothie is designed to refresh and rejuvenate you on a hot day. It makes use of a cucumber and a coconut - two of the most water-rich fruits that will not only nourish you but will hydrate your body as well. Add a banana, some leafy greens, a little bit of pineapple and the twist of ginger and you'll get a flavorful, nutrient-rich smoothie that will keep you wanting more.

What you need:

1 1/2 cups coconut water

1/4 cucumber

1 small ripe banana

1 rib celery

1 small handful parsley

1 cup fresh or frozen pineapple slices

1/2-inch ginger

6. Classic Strawberries and Cream

If you're a fan of the strawberries and cream combination, then this is one of the smoothie recipes for beginners that you can't afford to miss. Aside from being delicious, strawberries are chock full of Vitamin C that will help boost your energy. Bananas on the other hand are known to give any smoothie a delightful creamy texture. Drink this classic smoothie for breakfast to help jump start your energy for the rest of the day!

What you need:

1 cup fresh or frozen strawberries

1 small ripe banana

1/4 ripe avocado

1 1/2 cups unsweetened almond milk

1 tsp. vanilla extract

3-4 ice cubes

7. Green is In

If you're looking for low-calorie smoothie recipes, this is a good recipe to start with. Leafy greens aren't considered superfoods for nothing - they are low in calories but extremely rich in essential nutrients. If you're not fond of eating leafy greens, the apple and lemon both help neutralize the taste of this delicious smoothie.

What you need:

1 small head Romaine lettuce, chopped

1 1/2 cups chopped spinach

3 stalks celery

1 red apple, cored and chopped

Juice of 1/2 lemon

8. The Healthy Cooler

By using a variety of vegetables for your smoothie recipes for beginners, you will gain different vitamins and minerals that will help maintain your body's health. Concoct this deliciously nutritious smoothie to ensure both your mind and body's wellness.

What you need:

1 bunch spinach

1 handful parsley

4 stalks celery

2 large lettuce leaves

1 handful mint leaves

1 tbsp. fresh lemon juice

1/2-inch ginger

5 ice cubes

9. Berry Nutritious

Rich in vitamins, minerals and antioxidants, this mix is definitely one of the best smoothie recipes for beginners. With a delicious taste and an appetizing texture, this power smoothie will easily become one of your favorites!

What you need:

1 cup fresh or frozen mixed berries (strawberries, blueberries, raspberries, or blackberries)

1 cup oat milk

1 cup coconut milk

2 tsp. flaxseed

2 tbsp. organic natural yogurt

5-6 ice cubes

10. Classic Strawberry Smoothie

The Classic Strawberry smoothie is a popular breakfast choice. It's creamy, citrus-infused mix will jumpstart your energy levels at the beginning of the day and will also keep your tummy filled until lunchtime. Definitely a strawberry smoothie to try!

What you need:

6 frozen strawberries

1 medium banana

1 cup plain non-fat yogurt

1/2 cup freshly-squeezed orange juice

3-4 ice cubes

11. Strawberry-Kiwi Combo

Rich in Vitamin C and polyphenols, this strawberry smoothie is designed to help fight off diseases and keep your health in check. This delicious high-fiber concoction also helps curb your cravings and keep you feeling full longer. One of the best healthy smoothie recipes that helps you lose weight!

What you need:

5 fresh or frozen strawberries

1/2 ripe banana

1 small kiwi fruit, sliced

1 1/4 cups fresh apple juice

1 1/2 tsp. honey

3-4 ice cubes

3. All Berries Mix

Like strawberries, other berries such as blueberries, raspberries and blackberries are rich in essential nutrients, fiber and antioxidants. Boost your energy and promote healthy weight loss with a glass of this delightful berry fusion!

What you need:

3-4 frozen strawberries

1/2 cup berry mix (blueberries, raspberries, blackberries)

1/2 cup low-fat yogurt (any flavor)

Juice of 2 limes

3-4 ice cubes

12. Lumpy Strawberry Delight

Worried about your sugar intake? This sugar-free strawberry smoothie is a must try! It's rich in vitamins, minerals and protein that will instantly boost your energy. Turn a bad day around with this irresistible healthy smoothie recipe!

What you need:

1 cup fresh or frozen unsweetened strawberries

1 cup skim milk

1 tbsp. pumpkin or sunflower seeds

1 tbsp. cold-pressed organic flaxseed oil

13. Tropical Strawberry Splash

One of the most flavorful healthy smoothie recipes around, this filling smoothie mix makes a good post-workout drink. It's extremely hydrating, refreshing and energizing - not to mention mouth-watering!

What you need:

1/2 cup frozen strawberries

2 small ripe bananas, sliced

1/2 cup pineapple slices

1/2 cup fresh lemon juice

1/2 cup plain yogurt

3-4 ice cubes

14. Banana with a Twist

Monkeys don't love bananas for nothing - bananas are one of the healthiest, most delicious fruits around. They are rich in Vitamin B6, Vitamin C, potassium, manganese, copper and fiber which makes them a choice ingredient in fruit smoothie recipes. Along with the twist of ginger, this creamy smoothie mix is designed to help soothe stomach and digestive problems, heartburn and nausea. Definitely a treat you can't afford to miss!

What you need:

1 medium banana, sliced

1/2 tsp. freshly grated ginger

3/4 cup vanilla yogurt

1 tbsp. fresh honey

3-4 ice cubes

15. Creamy Citrus Treat

One of the best healthy fruit smoothies, this delicious low-calorie drink is designed to help you cool down on a hot day or after an intense workout. Citrus fruits like the orange are an excellent source of Vitamin C which helps boost energy and provides the body with plenty of health benefits.

What you need:

1 orange, peeled

2 tbsp. fresh lime juice

1/4 tsp. vanilla extract

1/4 cup fat-free yogurt

4 ice cubes

16. Blueberry-Green Tea Delight

This nutrient-dense fruit and tea smoothie is another popular choice in healthy fruit smoothies. Blueberries are rich in vitamins and antioxidants which help protect the body's cells from free radical damage. Green tea on the other hand hydrates and replenishes the body. Together, they make a delicious and refreshing smoothie!

What you need:

1 1/2 cup fresh or frozen blueberries

1 bag green tea

1/2 medium banana

2 tsp. honey

3/4 cup vanilla soy milk

3 tbsp. purified water

17. Pineapple Potion

When it comes to refreshing fruit smoothie recipes, this delicious mix is something you have to try. Pineapples are excellent sources of Vitamins A and C, calcium, phosphorus, potassium and fiber. They are known to help fight cough and colds, improve digestion and decrease the risk of macular degeneration among other things.

What you need:

1 cup pineapple chunks

1 cup low-fat vanilla yogurt

6 ice cubes

18. Mad About Mangoes

Mangoes are chock full of essential vitamins and minerals that some people refer to them as the "king of fruits". This delicious fleshy fruit is known for health benefits such as lowering cholesterol, alkalizing the body, preventing cancer, clearing the skin, improving eye function and so much more! This is one of the best fruit smoothie recipes you can drink for breakfast.

What you need:

2 ripe mangoes, peeled and chopped

6 apricots, peeled, pitted

1 cup plain low-fat yogurt

2 tsp. fresh lemon juice

1/4 tsp. vanilla extract

8 ice cubes

19. Strawberry & Banana Breakfast Smoothie

1 cup skim milk

3/4 cup low-fat yogurt

1/2 cup silken tofu

1 small banana

1-1/4 cups strawberries, preferably frozen

1/2 cup crushed ice

20. Blueberry & Banana Smoothie

1 cup skim milk

3/4 cup low-fat yogurt

1/2 cup silken tofu

1 banana, peeled and sliced

3/4 cup blueberries

1/2 cup crushed ice

21. Banana Smoothie

2 ripe bananas, peeled and sliced (preferably frozen)

1/4 cup low-fat vanilla or fruit yogurt

2 cups low-fat milk

2 tbsp wheat germ or oat bran

Ground nutmeg to taste (optional)

22. Mixed Berry Smoothie

1 cup frozen berries of your choice

1/4 cup low fat vanilla yogurt

1 tbsp malted milk powder

2 tsp wheat germ or oat bran

1 egg or egg substitute (optional)

23. Green Smoothie for Diabetics

2 cups water

2-3 cups lightly packed baby spinach leaves (preferably organic)

1 pear

1/2 to 1 banana

1/4 tsp cardamom

1-2 tbsp chia seeds (soak in 2 cups water for a while)

TIP: Chia seeds are high in fiber, calcium, protein, antioxidants and omega-3. You can buy them at health stores.

24. Strawberry Flax Smoothie

1 cup fresh or frozen strawberries

1/2 cup nonfat vanilla yogurt

1/2 cup skim milk

3 tbsp flax meal

1/2 tsp cinnamon

25. Cantaloupe Smoothies

Cantaloupe gives a subtle sweetness to any smoothie. It blends very well with citrus fruits. Don't stop there. Cantaloupe can mix deliciously with a variety of fruits.

A trick with using cantaloupe is to use ripe, juicy melons in order to use as little water as possible. This will create a smoothie bursting with flavor.

26. Orange Cantaloupe Smoothie

1/4 cantaloupe, large and ripe

1 orange, peeled and seeded

1 banana, frozen

5 ice cubes

1/2 teaspoon stevia

Place all of the fresh ingredients closest to the blade with the frozen ingredients on top. Blend until smooth. Serves 1-2

27. Lemon Smoothies

Another interesting fruit to use in your healthy fruit smoothies is a lemon. You can add a little zing to any smoothie recipe by using a half or whole peeled and seeded lemon. You can even use part of the peeling for a super strong lemon smoothie.

But brace yourself... The peeling makes a powerful smoothie! The lemon flavor might blast you over.

28. Lemon-Head Smoothie

1 lemon, peeled and seeded

1 banana, frozen

1 tsp stevia

1/2 cup water

3 ice cubes

Blend the lemon with the water. Add the banana, stevia, and ice and blend again. Serves 1

29. Mocha Smoothie:

8 ounces non-fat milk or soy milk

2 Tablespoons Herbalife Vanilla Formula 1 Soy Protein Smoothie Mix

½ teaspoon Decaffeinated Instant Coffee

4 - 6 ice cubes (optional)

Stir or blend in blender

30. Black Forest Smoothie

8 ounces non-fat milk or soy milk

2 Tablespoons Herbalife Chocolate Formula 1 Soy Protein Smoothie Mix

½ Teaspoon Black Walnut Extract

½ Banana (optional)

4-6 ice cubes (optional)

Stir or blend in blender

31. Citrus and Greens Delight

One piece of orange is equal to 59 calories. When you think about it, there are more fruits or vegetables that have a lower calorie count than an orange. But what makes it a great ingredient for healthy smoothie recipes for weight loss is its rich fiber content. According to a recent research from Australia, oranges top the list of fruits that are most filling. Add some low-calorie superfoods like leafy greens to the mix and you'll have a delicious glass of a fat-burning smoothie.

What you need:

2 oranges, peeled and seeded

1 small red apple

1 bunch baby spinach, chopped

3 large Romaine lettuce leaves

2 stalks celery

1 cup purified water

32. Be Berry Fit

Like other berries, blueberries are considered to be superfoods. These tiny, delicious fruits are excellent sources of essential vitamins and minerals. They are also rich in powerful antioxidants that help keep the body healthy. 1 serving of blueberries contains 4 grams of fiber which will help you feel full longer and will effectively suppress your appetite. This sweet fruit and vegetable mix is definitely one of the best smoothies for weight loss!

What you need:

2 cups fresh or frozen blueberries

1 large banana

2 tbsp. hemp seed, hulled

5 leaves kale

2 1/2 cups purified water

33. Apple-Dandelion Slimmer

If you're looking for healthy smoothie recipes for weight loss, you should look for one that uses an apple as an ingredient. Apples are one of the best fruits that aids in weight loss for plenty of reasons. For one, it contains a soluble fiber called pectin which helps block the absorption of bad cholesterol in the body. As a result, fat is utilized in the body instead of being stored. The fiber-rich peel of apples contains ursolic acid which according to a recent study, helps lower the risk of obesity.

What you need:

2 large apples

1 banana

1 bunch dandelion greens

1 lemon, peeled

2 tsp. flax seeds

4-5 ice cubes

CONCLUSION

CHOOSING THE BEST BLENDER FOR YOUR BUDGET

Again, when making a whole food Health Smoothie, DO NOT use a juicer, use a BLENDER! The best blender to use for a whole food Smoothie is a Vitamix, Bosch or K-tech. They are high-quality blenders and they come with a large container that can hold up to 60 ounces. They have a strong motor that lasts for years and save time because they quickly liquefy the mixture of vegetables, hard carrots, fruit and supplements. A high-power blender has a strong enough motor to actually blend and retain the fiber.

These high-quality blenders are investments in the $430 range, and the savings created by using a blender instead of a juicer are enormous when you consider the fact that no food volume is wasted, not to mention the decrease in health care costs which will be created by your new levels of health and energy.

Affordable and powerful blenders

You may also buy a simple blender at WalMart or most drug stores for between $39 and $89. These blenders work fine, provided they have a motor with at least 425-watts or more, so that they are strong enough to blend vegetables. A blender with a weak motor may not survive daily whole food Smoothies, so it's best to get a blender that has at least a 425-watt motor. Also, most of these less expensive units come with a container that is 40 oz instead of 60 oz. If the blender has a small pitcher (less than 40 oz), you may have to blend two batches instead of one.

I use an Oster or a Hamilton Beach for my travel blender. There are various blenders that are probably just as good, as long as they have a strong motor. I take my less expensive blender with me on the road and it fits in the trunk of my car or in my suitcase when I travel.

TIPS FOR FAST AND EFFICIENT BLENDING

You must have a blended drink on a daily basis to gain the maximum benefits from the whole foods. I know you can be successful if you follow these steps:

o Set your blender on the kitchen counter top, ready to use at all times rather than stored in a cabinet where you may forget about it. Human nature is such that if you see the blender ready to go, it is more likely that you will use it.

o Have a cutting board ready for some minor preparation to cut, remove stems and seeds or clean vegetables and fruit.

o Use sufficient water, soy or rice milk and ice in the drink so the consistency comes out smooth. The water line should come up to over half or three fourths of the blender line for proper blending of all the harder chunks of vegetables.

o The moment you pour out the blended concoction, immediately rinse the blender and any cutting utensils with fresh, hot water. Vegetables, fruit and sprouts easily rinse with water down the disposal after blending. However, if you wait to clean the blender pitcher later with the rest of the dishes, the thick, almost caked-on layer of vegetable matter will be much harder to clean. The common excuse of not wanting to "do the dishes" may give you a false reason to not want to blend again.

The whole process from putting vegetables, fruit and water in the blender to pouring out the completed drink, to rinsing the pitcher and utensils can be done in less than eight minutes - the time you would usually take to brew some coffee in the morning. If you don't have time to blend in the morning, then blend in the afternoon or evening. The key is that you do it on a daily basis to gain the youth-extending benefits of fat loss, increased energy and total body hydration.

www.ingramcontent.com/pod-product-compliance
Lightning Source LLC
Chambersburg PA
CBHW071124240526
45465CB00023B/801